EMBRACING MOTHERHOOD

A Comprehensive Guide To Newborn Care And Self Care

RUTH PETERS

COPYRIGHT

Copyright © 2023 Ruth Peters

TABLE OF CONTENT

INTRODUCTION

Congratulations on the beautiful journey of motherhood! The birth of your precious little one has brought immense joy, love, and a whirlwind of emotions into your life. As you embark on this incredible chapter, it's essential to equip yourself with knowledge and understanding to provide the best care for your newborn while prioritizing your own well-being.

"Embracing Motherhood: A Comprehensive Guide to Newborn Care and Self-Care" is here to support and empower you during this transformative period. This book has been lovingly crafted with the intention of providing you with practical advice, expert insights, and heartfelt encouragement, ensuring that you navigate this new world with confidence and grace.

Chapter by chapter, we will delve into the crucial aspects of newborn care, helping you understand the unique needs of your little one and guiding you through each milestone, from those early sleepless nights to establishing a nurturing routine. We will explore topics such as feeding and nutrition, diapering and hygiene, comforting techniques, and fostering a strong bond with your baby.

However, this book goes beyond newborn care. We acknowledge that your own well-being is just as important as your baby's, and we firmly believe that by nurturing yourself, you will become an even better mother. We will dive into the world of self-care, exploring strategies to prioritize your physical and mental health, manage the demands of motherhood, and embrace the joyous moments of this transformative journey.

Every mother's journey is unique, and there is no one-size-fits-all approach. Embracing Motherhood aims to be your trusted companion, supporting you through the ups and downs, guiding you with evidence-based information, and providing reassurance during moments of uncertainty.

As you navigate the challenges and triumphs of motherhood, always remember that you are not alone. You are part of a vast community of mothers who have walked this path before you and those who walk alongside you. Embracing Motherhood is a testament to the power of women supporting one another, and it is our hope that this book will serve as a guiding light, instilling you with confidence, resilience, and an unwavering love for both your baby and yourself.

Together, let's embark on this beautiful journey of motherhood, embracing the incredible role you now play and celebrating the bond that will grow stronger each day. Welcome to "Embracing Motherhood: A Comprehensive Guide to Newborn Care and Self-Care."

CHAPTER 1

EMBRACING THE ARRIVAL OF YOUR NEWBORN

Becoming a new mum is an incredible and transformative experience. It's normal to feel a mix of emotions, ranging from excitement and joy to anxiety and exhaustion. Embracing the arrival of your newborn involves finding balance, nurturing yourself, and creating a loving environment for your baby. Here are some tips to help you navigate this precious time:

Give yourself time to adjust: It's essential to acknowledge that adjusting to motherhood takes time. Be patient with yourself as you learn to care for your baby and adapt to your new role. Remember, it's okay to ask for help and seek support from loved ones or professionals.

Bond with your baby: Building a strong bond with your newborn is crucial for their development and your emotional connection. Spend quality time with your baby through activities like cuddling, skin-to-skin contact, gentle massages, and talking or singing to them. These moments will help you and your baby form a deep connection.

Prioritize self-care: Taking care of yourself is equally important as caring for your baby. Ensure you get enough time to rest, eat balanced, nutritious meals, and stay hydrated. Accept help from others, whether it's with household chores or looking after the baby, so you can have some time for yourself to relax and recharge.

Establish a routine: While newborns often have unpredictable schedules, establishing a flexible routine can provide a sense of structure and stability. Create a schedule for feeding, sleeping, and playtime that suits you and your baby's needs. Having a routine can help both of you feel more settled and comfortable.

Seek support and connect with other moms: Surround yourself with a supportive network of family, friends, and other moms who can offer guidance, empathy, and encouragement. Joining local parenting groups, attending mother-baby classes, or engaging in online communities can provide a sense of belonging and a platform to share experiences.

Embrace the small moments: Parenthood is filled with countless small but significant moments. Take the time to appreciate the little things, like your baby's first smile, their tiny fingers and toes, or the peaceful moments spent together. Embracing these precious moments can help you cherish the journey of motherhood.

Trust your instincts: Remember that you know your baby best. Trust your instincts and intuition when it comes to making decisions about their care. As you spend more time with your little one, you will become attuned to their needs and preferences.

Be gentle with yourself: It's natural to make mistakes or feel overwhelmed at times. Remember that being a mum is a learning process, and no one is perfect. Be gentle with yourself, practice self-compassion, and celebrate your accomplishments, no matter how small they may seem.

Capture memories: Time flies, and before you know it, your baby will grow up. Take plenty of photos, write down special moments in a journal, or create keepsakes to commemorate this beautiful chapter in your life. You will live to treasure these memories

Enjoy the journey: Embrace the arrival of your newborn by embracing the journey of motherhood itself. Every stage of your baby's growth is unique and filled with wonder. Embrace the ups and downs, the challenges and triumphs, and savor the joy that comes from nurturing and watching your little one grow.

FIRST MOMENT WITH YOUR NEWBORN

The first moments with your newborn are incredibly precious and form the foundation of your journey together. Here's an educational guide to help you navigate and make the most of those initial moments:

Skin-to-skin contact: Immediately after birth, practice skin-to-skin contact by placing your baby on your bare chest. This promotes bonding, regulates their body temperature, stabilizes heart rate, and enhances breastfeeding initiation.

First breastfeeding session: Initiate breastfeeding within the first hour, if possible. Seek guidance from lactation consultants or nurses to ensure proper latch and positioning. Remember, breastfeeding is a learning process for both you and your baby, so be patient and seek support as needed.

A gentle examination: Soon after birth, your baby will undergo a routine examination by a healthcare provider. This includes assessing vital signs, checking for any immediate health concerns, and performing standard tests and measurements.

Cord care: Follow the guidance of your healthcare provider regarding cord care. Keep the area clean and dry, avoiding submerging it in water until it has completely dried and detached (This will be discussed later in this book). Monitor for any signs of infection and consult your healthcare provider if you have concerns.

Diapering and dressing: Learn the basics of diapering your baby, including how to clean and change diapers (This will be discussed in details later in this book) Dress your baby in comfortable and weather-appropriate clothing. Remember to support their head and limbs while handling them.

Baby's first bath: Your healthcare provider will advise you on when and how to give your baby their first bath. Be gentle, use warm water, and choose mild, baby-friendly products. Maintain a secure grip while bathing, ensuring their safety at all times.

Soothing techniques: Babies may cry during their first moments as they adjust to the new environment. Try different soothing techniques, such as swaddling, gentle rocking, shushing sounds, or offering a pacifier. Respond to your baby's needs with love and patience.

Engaging with your newborn: Interact with your baby through eye contact, talking, and gentle touch. Sing lullabies, read books, and introduce them to the sound of your voice. These interactions foster emotional bonding and stimulate their developing senses.

Rest and recovery: Remember to prioritize your own rest and recovery during these first moments. Accept help from your partner, family, or friends to ensure you have enough time to rest, heal, and bond with your baby.

Each baby is unique, and there is no one-size-fits-all approach. Trust your instincts, seek guidance when needed, and embrace the joy and wonder of these first moments with your newborn. They mark the beginning of an incredible bond and a lifetime of love and learning together.

TAKING CARE OF YOURSELF

Taking care of yourself is crucial during the postpartum period as you recover from childbirth and adjust to the demands of motherhood. Let's look at tips to help you prioritize self-care and promote your postpartum recovery

1. Rest and sleep: Sleep deprivation is common for new moms, but getting enough rest is vital for your physical and mental well-being. Nap when your baby sleeps, and enlist the help of your partner or support system to share the responsibilities of nighttime feedings. Prioritize restorative sleep to aid your body's healing process.

2. Proper nutrition: Focus on nourishing your body with a balanced diet. Include nutrient-rich foods like fruits, vegetables, whole grains, lean proteins, and healthy fats. Stay hydrated by drinking plenty of water. If you're breastfeeding, consult a healthcare professional for specific dietary recommendations to support lactation.

3. Pain management: It's normal to experience some pain and discomfort after childbirth. Take prescribed pain medications as directed by your healthcare provider and use over-the-counter remedies such as ice packs, warm compresses, or sitz baths to

alleviate discomfort. Follow your healthcare provider's instructions for managing any specific postpartum pain or concerns.

4. Pelvic floor exercises: Strengthening your pelvic floor muscles is essential for recovery, especially if you've had a vaginal delivery. Perform gentle pelvic floor exercises, commonly known as Kegels, to improve muscle tone and prevent urinary incontinence. Consult a healthcare provider or a pelvic floor therapist for proper guidance on performing these exercises.

5. Gradual physical activity: Ease into physical activity gradually, based on your healthcare provider's guidance. Begin with gentle walks and gradually increase your activity level over time. Physical activity can boost your mood, increase energy levels, and promote overall well-being. Listen to your body and don't push yourself beyond your limits.

6. Emotional well-being: The postpartum period can bring a range of emotions, including baby blues or postpartum depression. Prioritize your emotional well-being by seeking support from loved ones, joining support groups, or speaking with a therapist. Share your feelings openly and don't hesitate to ask for help when needed.

7. Body image and self-acceptance: Embrace the changes in your body and give yourself grace during the postpartum period.

Remember that it took time for your body to grow and birth a baby, and it will take time to heal and recover. Focus on self-acceptance and celebrate the incredible feat your body has accomplished.

8. Time for yourself: Carve out moments for self-care and personal time. Engage in activities that bring you joy, whether it's taking a relaxing bath, reading a book, practicing mindfulness or meditation, or pursuing a hobby. Prioritize self-care as it will replenish your energy and help you better care for your baby.

9. Reach out for support: Don't hesitate to ask for help or support from your partner, family, friends, or healthcare professionals. Surround yourself with a supportive network that can lend a helping hand, provide guidance, and offer emotional support during this transformative period.

10.   Celebrate milestones: Acknowledge and celebrate your postpartum milestones, whether big or small. Each day, week, or month that passes is a testament to your strength and resilience as a new mother. Take pride in the progress you make and cherish the journey of postpartum recovery.

You should know that, self-care is not selfish—it's an essential part of being a healthy and happy mom. By prioritizing your own well-being, you'll be better equipped to care for and nurture your baby. Embrace self-compassion, be patient with yourself, and celebrate the beautiful journey of postpartum recovery.

CHAPTER 2

UNDERSTANDING YOUR BABY

Understanding your newborn's appearance, reflexes, and senses can help you better connect with and care for your baby. Here's a guide to help you navigate and appreciate these aspects of your newborn's development:

Appearance:

Understanding your baby's appearance can provide valuable insights into their health and development. Here are some key aspects of a newborn's appearance that can help you understand your baby better:

1. Head shape: Newborns often have slightly misshapen heads due to the pressures of birth. The shape usually evens out over time as the baby grows. However, if you notice any unusual or persistent abnormalities, consult your pediatrician.
2. Fontanelles: Fontanelles are the soft spots on a baby's head where the skull bones haven't fused yet. There are typically two fontanelles: a larger one at the top of the head and a smaller one toward the back. These soft spots allow for brain growth and provide flexibility during birth. Be cautious when touching them and avoid applying pressure.

3. Hair: Newborns' hair can vary greatly. Some babies are born with a full head of hair, while others have very little or no hair at all. Hair color and texture can change as your baby grows, so don't be surprised if it undergoes transformation.

4. Eyes: Your baby's eye color may change over time. Many newborns have bluish-gray or dark-colored eyes initially, but the final eye color may not be apparent until several months or even years later. Additionally, it's common for newborns' eyes to appear crossed or wander occasionally. This is typically due to their developing eye muscles and should resolve naturally.

5. Skin color and complexion: Newborns' skin can range from pink to red, and sometimes even have a yellowish tinge known as jaundice. Jaundice is usually harmless and fades away on its own within a few weeks. Some babies may have temporary skin conditions like milia (tiny white bumps), baby acne, or peeling skin, which are normal and tend to resolve without treatment.

6. Facial features: Newborns often have round faces with full cheeks. Their facial features may appear puffy due to fluid retention or birth-related molding. As your baby grows, their facial structure will become more defined.

7. Hands and feet: Your baby's hands and feet may appear bluish or cool to the touch in the first few days. This is normal and usually resolves as their circulation improves. Additionally, newborns often have long, slender fingers and toes with soft, flexible nails. Be cautious when trimming their nails to avoid accidentally cutting their delicate skin.

Reflexes:

Understanding your baby's reflexes can help you interpret their behaviors and responses. Reflexes are automatic, involuntary movements or actions that are present from birth. Here are some common reflexes seen in newborns:

1. Rooting reflex: When you stroke your baby's cheek or corner of their mouth, they will turn their head in that direction and open their mouth in search of a nipple or a source of food. This reflex helps with breastfeeding or bottle-feeding.
2. Sucking reflex: When an object touches the roof of your baby's mouth or their lips, they will instinctively start sucking. This reflex is essential for feeding and can often be seen during breastfeeding or bottle-feeding.
3. Grasping reflex: If you place your finger or an object in your baby's palm or near their fingers, they will automatically close their hand around it. This reflex helps them hold onto objects and is an early step toward developing intentional grasping.
4. Moro reflex: Also known as the startle reflex, this occurs when your baby is startled by a sudden noise, movement, or sensation. They will throw their arms and legs outward, arch their back, and then bring their arms back in a hugging motion. This reflex is thought to be a protective response and usually diminishes by the third or fourth month.
5. Stepping reflex: If you hold your baby upright with their feet touching a solid surface, they will mimic stepping movements, making it appear as though they are trying to walk. This reflex is not actual walking but rather an automatic response and usually disappears after a few weeks.
6. Babinski reflex: When you stroke the sole of your baby's foot from the heel towards the toes, their toes will fan out and their

big toe will extend upward. This reflex is normal in infants and indicates a healthy neurological development.

7. Tonic neck reflex: If you turn your baby's head to one side, the arm on that side will extend and the opposite arm bends at the elbow. It usually disappears around 4-6 months of age.

8. Blinking and cough reflexes: Newborns have automatic reflexes like blinking to protect their eyes from bright lights or foreign objects, and coughing or gagging when their airway is stimulated. These reflexes help keep your baby safe.

It's important to note that reflexes vary from baby to baby, and they can change or disappear as your baby grows. They are a normal part of development and usually don't require any intervention. However, if you have concerns about your baby's reflexes or notice any unusual or absent reflexes, it's advisable to discuss them with your pediatrician during regular check-ups.

Senses

Understanding your newborn's senses can help you better engage and nurture their development. Although their senses are still developing, newborns are capable of perceiving and responding to the world around them. Here's an overview of your baby's senses:

1. Vision: At birth, a newborn's vision is quite limited. They can see objects and people at close distances (about 8-12 inches) most clearly. Their vision is best in high-contrast colors, such as black and white or bold, contrasting colors. Over time, their visual acuity improves, and they start to track moving objects and focus on faces

2. Hearing: Newborns have a well-developed sense of hearing. They can recognize familiar voices, especially that of their parents, and are sensitive to sounds and noises in their environment. Soft, gentle sounds and soothing lullabies can be comforting to them. Be mindful of loud or sudden noises, as they may startle your baby.

3. Smell: A newborn's sense of smell is highly developed from birth. They can recognize the scent of their mother's breast milk, which helps facilitate breastfeeding. Babies may also have preferences for certain smells, such as the familiar scent of their parents. Pleasant and comforting smells, such as those from their mother or a familiar blanket, can have a calming effect.

4. Taste: Newborns have taste preferences even before birth. They can differentiate between sweet, bitter, and sour tastes. Breast milk and formula provide different tastes, and your baby may have preferences for one over the other. It's important to note that solid foods are typically introduced around 4-6 months of age.

5. Touch: The sense of touch is highly developed in newborns. They can feel and respond to different textures, temperatures, and pressures. Gentle touches, massages, and skin-to-skin contact are not only comforting but also help with bonding and attachment. Providing your baby with a variety of safe and tactile experiences can stimulate their sense of touch.

6. Proprioception: Proprioception refers to a baby's awareness of their body position and movement. Even as newborns, they have a sense of their body's orientation and can detect changes in position. Swaddling, being held, or placed in different positions can help them feel secure and comfortable.

7. Vestibular sense: The vestibular sense is responsible for maintaining balance and spatial orientation. Newborns have a rudimentary sense of balance, but it rapidly develops in the first year. Gentle rocking, being carried, or experiencing gentle movements can be soothing for your baby and promote their vestibular development.

Remember, each baby develops at their own pace. If you have concerns about your baby's appearance, reflexes, or sensory responses, consult your healthcare provider for guidance and reassurance. Enjoy this special time of getting to know your baby and witnessing their growth and development.

CHAPTER 3

FEEDING YOUR BABY

BREASTFEEDING

Breastfeeding is a wonderful way to nourish and bond with your baby. This method of feeding your baby offers numerous benefits for both the mother and the baby.

Here's a guide to help you understand the basics of breastfeeding:

Positioning and Latching: Find a comfortable and quiet place to breastfeed your baby. Support your back with pillows if needed. Position your baby so that their whole body is facing you, with their head in line with your breast. Ensure that their nose is level with your nipple. When your baby opens their mouth wide, bring them in close, aiming their bottom lip well below the nipple. The latch should be deep, with your baby's mouth covering a large portion of the areola (the darker area around the nipple). A good latch is important for effective breastfeeding and minimizing discomfort.

Establishing a Milk Supply: During the first few days after birth, your body produces colostrum, a nutrient-rich fluid that provides essential antibodies and nutrients for your baby. Colostrum is produced in small quantities but is highly concentrated. It gradually transitions to mature milk within a week or so. Frequent and on-demand breastfeeding in the early days helps establish your milk supply. Ensure that your baby nurses from both breasts during each feeding session.

Feeding on Demand: Breastfed babies often need to nurse frequently, as breast milk is digested more quickly than formula. Watch for hunger cues such as rooting, sucking motions, or putting hands to the mouth. Aim for at least 8-12 nursing sessions in 24 hours. Feeding on demand helps establish a good milk supply and ensures your baby is getting enough nourishment.

Signs of Adequate Feeding: Your baby is getting enough milk if they have a good latch, nurse for 10-15 minutes or longer on each breast, and have a satisfied appearance after feeding. They should produce several wet diapers (at least 6-8) per day and have regular bowel movements. Weight gain and growth in length and head circumference are also signs of adequate feeding.

Proper Breast Care: Keep your breasts clean and dry. Avoid using soap on your nipples as it can dry out the skin. After each feeding, express a few drops of breast milk and gently rub it onto your nipples to help soothe and protect them. If you experience discomfort or soreness, consult a lactation consultant or healthcare provider for guidance.

Breastfeeding Positions: There are various breastfeeding positions you can try to find what works best for you and your baby. Some common positions include the cradle hold, cross-cradle hold, football hold, and side-lying position. Experiment with different positions to find the one that is comfortable and allows your baby to latch well.

Breast Pumping and Storing Milk: If you need to express milk or build up a supply, you can use a breast pump. There are different types of pumps available, including manual and electric options. Follow the manufacturer's instructions for proper usage. Expressed milk can be stored in sterilized containers in the refrigerator for up to 4-6 days or in the freezer for several months. Be sure to label the containers with the date.

Seek Support: Breastfeeding can sometimes be challenging, especially in the early weeks. Seek support from a lactation consultant, breastfeeding support groups, or your healthcare provider. They can provide guidance, answer your questions, and offer assistance to help you overcome any difficulties you may encounter.

EXCLUSIVE BREASTFEEDING

Exclusive breastfeeding refers to feeding your baby only breast milk, without the addition of any other liquids or solid foods, for the first six months of their life. Here's some information to help you understand the benefits of exclusive breastfeeding:

1. Optimal Nutrition: Breast milk is uniquely designed to provide all the necessary nutrients, vitamins, and minerals your baby needs for healthy growth and development. It contains the perfect balance of proteins, fats, carbohydrates, and antibodies that protect against infections and diseases.

2. Immunological Benefits: Breast milk contains antibodies and immune-boosting substances that help protect your baby from various illnesses and infections, such as respiratory infections, ear infections, gastrointestinal infections, and allergies. The antibodies in breast milk help strengthen your baby's immune system and provide them with passive immunity.

3. Digestive Health: Breast milk is easily digested by your baby's immature digestive system. It reduces the likelihood of constipation and diarrhea, and it is less likely to cause digestive issues compared to formula feeding.

4. Cognitive Development: Breast milk contains essential fatty acids, such as DHA (docosahexaenoic acid), which are crucial for brain development and cognitive function. Studies have suggested that breastfeeding may have a positive impact on cognitive development and intelligence.

5. Bonding and Emotional Connection: Exclusive breastfeeding provides an opportunity for skin-to-skin contact, eye contact, and closeness with

your baby. These interactions promote bonding, emotional connection, and a sense of security for both you and your baby.

6. Reduced Risk of Chronic Conditions: Breastfeeding has been associated with a reduced risk of various chronic conditions in later life, including obesity, type 2 diabetes, asthma, allergies, and certain types of childhood cancers. Also for the mother, breastfeeding has been linked to a lower risk of breast cancer, ovarian cancer, and type 2 diabetes in mothers. It may also help lower the risk of postmenopausal osteoporosis.

7. Postpartum Recovery: Breastfeeding triggers the release of hormones that aid in the contraction of the uterus, helping it return to its pre-pregnancy size more quickly. It also helps reduce postpartum bleeding and may assist with weight loss.

8. Breast Milk Supply: The more you breastfeed, the more milk your body produces. Exclusive breastfeeding helps establish and maintain a good milk supply. Feeding on-demand and allowing your baby to nurse frequently ensures a healthy milk production.

9. Convenient and Cost-Effective: Breastfeeding is convenient as breast milk is always available at the right temperature, ready to nourish your baby. It eliminates the need for formula preparation, sterilization of bottles, and constant bottle feeding. Breastfeeding can also save you money by avoiding the cost of formula and feeding supplies.

10. Environmental Benefits: Breastfeeding is environmentally friendly as it produces no waste, requires no packaging, and has a minimal carbon footprint compared to formula feeding.

Exclusive breastfeeding is a personal choice, and it may not be feasible or suitable for everyone. The most important thing is to provide love, care, and nourishment for your baby in the way that works best for you and your family.

You should also note that every mother and baby are unique, and breastfeeding may not be possible or suitable for everyone. It's essential to make an informed decision based on your individual circumstances and consult with healthcare professionals for guidance and support. Whether you breastfeed exclusively, partially, or for a short period, any amount of breastfeeding can provide benefits for you and your baby.

FORMULA FEEDING

Formula feeding is a safe and viable option for nourishing your baby if breastfeeding is not possible, chosen, or a combination of breast milk and formula is preferred. Here are important things to know and keep in mind if you choose this method of feeding.

1. Types of Formula: Infant formula is available in various types, such as cow's milk-based formula, soy-based formula (for babies with lactose intolerance or cow's milk protein allergy), hydrolyzed formula (where the proteins are partially broken down), and specialized formulas for specific medical conditions. It's important

to choose a formula that is appropriate for your baby's needs. Consult with your healthcare provider for guidance in selecting the right formula.

2. Sterilization and Preparation: It is essential to maintain proper hygiene and cleanliness when preparing formula. Wash your hands thoroughly before handling formula and sterilize the bottles, nipples, and other feeding equipment according to the manufacturer's instructions. Follow the formula package instructions to ensure accurate measurements and appropriate water-to-formula ratios. Use water that has been boiled and cooled for formula preparation unless otherwise advised by your healthcare provider.

3. Feeding Schedule: Newborns typically need to be fed on-demand, following their hunger cues. As your baby grows, they may settle into a more predictable feeding schedule. Pay attention to your baby's cues for hunger and fullness, and avoid overfeeding or forcing them to finish a bottle.

4. Bonding and Connection: Although formula feeding may not involve direct breastfeeding, it provides an opportunity for bonding and closeness. Hold your baby close during feeding, make eye contact, and engage in gentle touches and soft, soothing sounds. These nurturing interactions help develop the emotional connection between you and your baby.

5. Burping: During bottle feeding, it is important to pause periodically to burp your baby. This helps release trapped air and reduces the likelihood of discomfort or gas. Hold your baby upright against your shoulder or sit them upright and gently pat or rub their back until they burp.

6. Cleaning and Storage: After each feeding, wash the bottles and nipples with warm soapy water, rinse thoroughly, and allow them to air dry or sanitize them according to the manufacturer's instructions. Prepared formula can be stored in the refrigerator for a limited time, usually up to 24 hours. Discard any unused formula left in the bottle after a feeding to prevent bacterial growth.

7. Transitioning: If you decide to transition from breastfeeding to formula feeding or introduce formula alongside breastfeeding, it can be done gradually. Slowly replace one breastfeeding session with a bottle of formula and gradually increase the number of formula feeds over time. This gradual transition helps both you and your baby adjust.

Remember, formula feeding can be a positive and nurturing experience for both you and your baby. Trust your instincts, follow safe preparation practices, and enjoy the bonding moments that come with feeding your little one.

COMBINING THE TWO OPTIONS

Combining breastfeeding and formula feeding, also known as mixed feeding or supplementation, can be a flexible approach that suits the needs of both you and your baby. Here's some information to help you navigate this approach:

1. Reasons for Combination Feeding: There are various reasons why a mother may choose to combine breastfeeding and formula feeding. It could be due to low milk supply, difficulties with breastfeeding, returning to work or other commitments, or personal preference. It's important to remember that any amount of breast milk you provide to your baby is beneficial.

2. Establishing Breastfeeding: If you plan to combine breastfeeding and formula feeding from the beginning, it's recommended to establish breastfeeding first before introducing formula. This allows you and your baby to develop a strong breastfeeding relationship and helps ensure a good milk supply. Breastfeed your baby frequently, on-demand, and seek support from a lactation consultant if needed.

3. Introducing Formula: When introducing formula, start by replacing one breastfeeding session with a bottle of formula. This can be done gradually, allowing your baby to adjust to the new feeding routine. Observe your baby's cues and respond accordingly. Over time, you can increase the number of formula feeds while continuing to breastfeed as much as you and your baby desire.

4. Choosing Formula: Select a formula that is suitable for your baby's age and nutritional needs. Consult with your healthcare provider if you have any concerns or if your baby has specific dietary requirements.

5. Pumping and Maintaining Milk Supply: If you plan to continue breastfeeding alongside formula feeding, it's important to pump breast milk regularly to maintain your milk supply. Pumping after formula feeds or during the times you would typically breastfeed can help stimulate milk production. Store the expressed milk in sterilized containers in the refrigerator or freezer for future use.

6. Feeding Schedule and Routines: Establish a feeding schedule that works for you and your baby. You can breastfeed during certain times of the day and offer formula feeds at other times. Alternatively, you can choose to breastfeed for some feeds and formula feed for others throughout the day. Find a routine that fits your lifestyle and allows you to provide both breast milk and formula as desired.

7. Bonding and Connection: Whether you breastfeed or formula feed, feeding time is an opportunity for bonding and connection. Maintain eye contact, hold your baby close, and engage in gentle touches and soothing sounds. These nurturing interactions promote a strong emotional connection between you and your baby.

FEEDING YOUR BABY AS A WORKING-CLASS MUM

Feeding your baby as a working-class mum can present unique challenges, but with careful planning and support, it's possible to provide nourishment for your baby while managing work responsibilities. Here are some tips to help you navigate feeding your baby as a working mum:

1. Plan Ahead: Before returning to work, start preparing for the transition by researching and understanding your options for feeding your baby. Decide whether you plan to breastfeed, pump breast milk, use formula, or a combination of these methods. Understanding your chosen approach will help you plan accordingly.

2. Breastfeeding and Pumping: If you choose to breastfeed, consider pumping and storing breast milk to ensure a supply for when you're away from your baby. Invest in a quality breast pump and practice pumping before you go back to work to become familiar with the process. Plan your pumping schedule and designate a comfortable and private space at work where you can express milk. Communicate with your employer about your pumping needs and work together to find a suitable arrangement.

3. Building a Milk Supply: Start building a freezer stash of breast milk before returning to work. Begin pumping a few extra times a day after feeding your baby to stimulate milk production and gradually build up your supply. Store expressed breast milk in labeled containers or bags in the freezer, following proper storage guidelines.

4. Pumping Routine: Establish a pumping routine that aligns with your work schedule. Aim to pump at regular intervals, typically every 3-4

hours, to maintain your milk supply and provide enough milk for your baby. Use a hands-free pumping bra to allow you to multitask while pumping, which can save time.

5. Feeding Schedule: Coordinate with your childcare provider to establish a feeding schedule that aligns with your work hours. Provide them with the necessary breast milk or formula, along with instructions on feeding quantities and preferences.

6. Formula Feeding: If you choose to formula feed, prepare bottles of formula in advance and store them in the refrigerator or bring pre-measured powdered formula to mix with water as needed. Make sure your childcare provider is familiar with your baby's feeding routine and preferences.

7. Meal Planning: As a working mum, you may find it helpful to plan and prepare meals and snacks in advance. Consider batch cooking or meal prepping on weekends to ensure you have nutritious meals readily available. A well-balanced diet will help maintain your energy levels and support breastfeeding if you choose to do so.

8. Seek Support: Reach out to your employer, colleagues, friends, and family for support and understanding. Inform them of your feeding goals and any accommodations you may need at work. Connect with other working mums who have gone through similar experiences for advice and encouragement.

9. Self-Care: Remember to prioritize self-care to manage the demands of work and caring for your baby. Take breaks, find time to relax, and get enough rest. Proper self-care will help you maintain your physical and mental well-being, which in turn supports your ability to provide for your baby.

10. Flexible Work Arrangements: Explore flexible work arrangements, if possible, such as adjusted schedules, remote work options, or on-site childcare facilities. These arrangements can facilitate easier breastfeeding or pumping sessions and provide more quality time with your baby.

It's important to remember that every working mum's situation is unique, and you should find a feeding approach that works best for you and your baby. With proper planning, open communication, and a support system in place, you can successfully navigate feeding your baby while managing your work responsibilities.

CHAPTER 4

SLEEPING AND SOOTHING

Understanding your newborn's sleep patterns can help you establish a healthy sleep routine and ensure your baby gets the rest they need. Here's some information to help you understand newborn sleep patterns:

Sleep Duration: Newborns sleep for varying durations throughout the day and night, typically ranging from 14 to 17 hours in a 24-hour period. However, they don't sleep for long stretches at a time and instead have shorter sleep cycles.

Sleep Cycles: Newborns have shorter sleep cycles compared to older children and adults. Their sleep cycles typically last around 40-60 minutes, and they go through multiple cycles throughout the day and night. During each sleep cycle, your baby will transition between light sleep, deep sleep, and active sleep.

Irregular Sleep: Newborns do not have a regular sleep pattern and often sleep in short bursts. They may sleep for a few minutes to a couple of hours before waking up. It's normal for their sleep to be unpredictable and inconsistent during the first few months.

Day-Night Confusion: Many newborns have difficulty differentiating between day and night. They may be more wakeful and alert during the night and sleepier during the day.

Hunger and Sleep: Newborns have small stomachs and require frequent feedings. They often wake up to feed every 2-3 hours, including during the night. Hunger cues are a common reason for their waking up. As your baby grows, they may start to sleep for longer stretches between feedings.

Sleep Associations: Newborns may develop sleep associations, such as being rocked, cuddled, or fed to sleep. These associations can help soothe your baby to sleep, but they may also rely on them to fall back asleep when they wake up during the night. Gentle techniques like creating a calm sleep environment and establishing consistent bedtime routines can help your baby learn healthy sleep habits.

Safety Guidelines: Ensure that your baby's sleep environment is safe to reduce the risk of Sudden Infant Death Syndrome (SIDS). Place your baby on their back to sleep on a firm mattress in a crib or bassinet, without pillows, blankets, or stuffed toys. Keep the room at a comfortable temperature and avoid overheating your baby.

Be Patient: Remember that newborn sleep patterns evolve over time. As your baby grows, they will gradually develop more predictable sleep cycles and longer periods of sleep. Be patient and understanding as you navigate their changing sleep patterns.

ESTABLISHING HEALTHY SLEEPING HABIT

Establishing healthy sleep habits in a newborn can take time and patience, but with consistent efforts, you can help your baby develop good sleep routines. Here are some tips to help you establish healthy sleeping habits in your newborn:

1. Create a Sleep-Friendly Environment: Set up a calm and comfortable sleep environment for your baby. Use a firm mattress and ensure the crib or bassinet meets safety guidelines. Keep the room dimly lit, maintain a comfortable temperature, and use white noise or soft music to create a soothing atmosphere.
2. Differentiate Day and Night: Help your baby understand the difference between day and night. During the day, expose your baby to natural light, engage in playtime, and keep the environment bright and stimulating. At night, create a calm and quiet atmosphere with minimal stimulation to promote sleep.
3. Establish a Bedtime Routine: Establishing a consistent bedtime routine signals to your baby that it's time to wind down and prepare for sleep. Start the routine with soothing activities such as a warm bath, gentle massage, quiet time, lullabies, or reading a bedtime story. Keep the routine calm, predictable, and consistent each night.
4. Observe Sleep Cues: Learn to recognize your baby's sleep cues, such as yawning, rubbing eyes, or becoming fussy. Respond promptly to these cues and initiate the bedtime routine when you notice them. Putting your baby to sleep when they are drowsy but still awake can help them learn to self-soothe and fall asleep independently.
5. Encourage Daytime Wakefulness: During the day, engage your baby in interactive play, tummy time, and social interactions to help them stay awake and active. Expose them to natural light and noise to reinforce the concept that daytime is for wakefulness and nighttime is for sleep.
6. Establish Regular Sleep Times: While newborns may not adhere to strict schedules, aim to establish regular sleep times by creating a

consistent routine around naps and bedtime. Over time, your baby's internal clock will begin to adjust to these patterns, making it easier for them to fall asleep and stay asleep.

7. Practice Safe Sleep: Follow safe sleep practices to reduce the risk of Sudden Infant Death Syndrome (SIDS). Place your baby on their back to sleep, ensure the sleep environment is free of hazards like loose bedding or stuffed animals, and avoid overheating.

8. Encourage Self-Soothing: As your baby grows, encourage them to self-soothe and fall asleep independently. Place your baby in the crib when they are drowsy but still awake, allowing them to learn how to settle themselves to sleep. This helps them develop self-regulation skills and reduces reliance on external sleep aids.

9. Be Consistent: Consistency is key when establishing healthy sleep habits. Stick to the established bedtime routine and sleep schedule as much as possible, even during weekends or holidays. Consistency helps your baby develop a sense of predictability and security around sleep.

SOOTHING A FUSSY BABY

When your baby becomes fussy or irritable, it can be challenging to figure out how to soothe them. Every baby is unique, so it may take some trial and error to find what works best for your little one. Here are some soothing techniques you can try:

1. Gentle Touch and Cuddling: Hold your baby close and provide gentle, rhythmic movements such as rocking, swaying, or

bouncing. The warmth and security of your touch can help calm and comfort them.

2. Skin-to-Skin Contact: Undress your baby and place them against your bare chest, allowing for skin-to-skin contact. This technique, also known as kangaroo care, can help regulate their body temperature, heart rate, and promote bonding and relaxation.

3. White Noise: Background noise, such as white noise, can mimic the sounds your baby heard in the womb and help soothe them. You can use a white noise machine, a fan, or even a smartphone app that provides calming sounds like ocean waves or rainfall.

4. Swaddling: Wrap your baby snugly in a lightweight blanket or a specially designed swaddle blanket. Swaddling can help your baby feel secure and limit their startle reflex, promoting better sleep and relaxation.

5. Sucking: Offer a pacifier, your clean finger, or let your baby nurse if you are breastfeeding. Sucking is a natural soothing mechanism for babies and can help calm them down.

6. Massage: Gently massage your baby's body using soft strokes and gentle pressure. You can use baby-safe oil or lotion to make the massage more soothing. Massaging their back, tummy, or feet can help relax their muscles and promote a sense of calm.

7. Change of Environment: Sometimes a change of scenery can distract and soothe a fussy baby. Take your baby for a walk outside, sit near a window with a view, or simply move to a different room to provide a change in sensory stimulation.

8. Gentle Motion: Experiment with different types of motion to see what your baby finds soothing. Some babies may respond well to being walked or strolled in a pram, while others may prefer a gentle ride in a car or a baby swing.

9. Calming Rituals: Establish calming rituals before sleep or during fussy periods. This could include dimming the lights, playing soft music, giving a gentle massage, or reading a bedtime story. Consistency and repetition will help signal to your baby that it's time to relax.

10. Stay Calm and Reassuring: Babies can pick up on your emotions, so it's important to stay calm and reassuring when trying to soothe them. Speak to your baby in a soothing tone, maintain a relaxed demeanor, and provide a comforting presence.

Remember that not all techniques will work for every baby, so it's essential to pay attention to your baby's cues and adjust your approach accordingly. Trust your instincts as a parent and be patient as you navigate the soothing process with your little one. If you're concerned about your baby's fussiness or if they continue to be inconsolable, it's always a good idea to consult with your pediatrician to rule out any underlying issues or medical conditions.

CHAPTER 5

HYGIENE

DIAPERING

Choosing the right diaper for your baby is important to ensure their comfort, prevent leaks, and maintain good skin health. Here are some factors to consider when selecting diapers:

1. Size: Diapers come in different sizes based on your baby's weight. It's important to choose the right size to ensure a proper fit. Diapers that are too small can be uncomfortable and may cause leaks, while diapers that are too large may not provide a secure fit and can also lead to leaks.

2. Absorbency: Look for diapers with good absorbency to keep your baby dry and prevent leaks. High-quality diapers often have a moisture-wicking layer that draws wetness away from your baby's skin, keeping them comfortable for longer periods.

3. Breathability: Opt for diapers that are breathable and allow air circulation. Breathable diapers help prevent diaper rash and keep your baby's skin healthy by reducing moisture build-up.

4. Softness: Choose diapers made from soft materials to ensure your baby's comfort. Diapers with a soft inner lining are gentle on your baby's delicate skin and help prevent irritation.

5. Stretchable and Flexible: Look for diapers with stretchable side panels and flexible waistbands. These features provide a snug fit while allowing your baby to move freely and comfortably.

6. Diaper Type: Decide whether you want to use disposable diapers or cloth diapers. Disposable diapers are convenient as they can be easily disposed of after use. Cloth diapers, on the other hand, are reusable and can be a cost-effective and eco-friendly option in the long run.

7. Allergies and Sensitivities: Consider any allergies or sensitivities your baby may have. Some babies have sensitive skin and may require hypoallergenic diapers that are free from fragrances, lotions, and other potential irritants.

8. Brand and Reviews: Research different diaper brands and read reviews from other parents to get an idea of their performance, reliability, and overall customer satisfaction. Personal recommendations from other parents can also be helpful.

It's worth noting that every baby is different, and what works well for one baby may not work for another. You may need to try different diaper brands and types to find the one that suits your baby best. Pay attention to your baby's comfort and skin health, and make adjustments as necessary.

Here are some essentials and tips to help a new mum with diapering:

1. Diapers: Stock up on an adequate supply of diapers in the appropriate size for your baby. Newborns typically start with newborn-sized diapers and then transition to larger sizes as they grow. You can choose between disposable diapers or cloth diapers, depending on your preference.

2. Wipes: Have a pack of baby wipes on hand for easy and gentle cleaning during diaper changes. Look for wipes that are specifically designed for sensitive baby skin and are free from harsh chemicals or fragrances.

3. Diaper Rash Cream: Diaper rash can occur, so it's helpful to have a diaper rash cream or ointment available. Apply a thin layer to clean and dry skin to create a protective barrier and soothe any irritation.

4. Changing Pad: A changing pad or mat provides a clean and comfortable surface for diaper changes. It helps protect your baby from coming into contact with any potentially dirty or unhygienic surfaces.

5. Diaper Pail or Diaper Disposal System: Consider using a diaper pail or a diaper disposal system to contain and lock away used diapers. These help to minimize odors and make diaper disposal more convenient.

6. Diaper Bag: Invest in a spacious and well-organized diaper bag to carry all the diapering essentials when you're on the go. Look for one with multiple compartments to keep things organized and easy to find.

7. Extra Clothing: Keep a few extra sets of baby clothes in your diaper bag or within reach during diaper changes. Sometimes accidents happen, and having spare clothing handy will save you from having to search for clean clothes in a hurry.

8. Diaper Changing Essentials: Have a supply of cotton balls or soft cloths for wiping, along with a diaper rash cream applicator if needed. You may also want to keep a small bottle of hand sanitizer or wipes to clean your hands after each diaper change.

9. Diapering Technique: When changing your baby's diaper, make sure to wash your hands before and after the diaper change. Lay your baby on the changing pad, remove the dirty diaper, and use wipes to clean the diaper area gently. Then, place a fresh diaper under your baby, secure it snugly but not too tight, and dispose of the soiled diaper appropriately.

PREVENTING DIAPER RASH

As a first-time mum, preventing diaper rash is an important aspect of your baby's skincare routine. Diaper rash is a common condition characterized by inflamed and irritated skin in the diaper area. While it's common and often not serious, it can be uncomfortable for your little one. Here are some tips to help you prevent diaper rash:

1. Change diapers frequently: Regularly changing your baby's diapers is crucial in preventing diaper rash. Wet or soiled diapers can irritate the skin, so aim to change them every two to three hours or as soon as you notice they are wet or soiled.

2. Clean the diaper area gently: During diaper changes, use a gentle, fragrance-free baby wipe or a soft cloth with warm water to clean your baby's diaper area. Avoid using harsh soaps, wipes with alcohol, or scented wipes, as these can be irritating to the skin.

3. Pat dry, don't rub: After cleaning the diaper area, pat it dry gently with a soft towel or allow it to air dry. Avoid rubbing the skin, as this can cause further irritation.

4. Use a barrier ointment or cream: Applying a thin layer of a diaper rash cream or ointment can create a protective barrier between your baby's skin and the diaper. Look for products that contain zinc oxide or petroleum jelly, as these ingredients help soothe and protect the skin.

5. Choose the right diapers: Opt for diapers that are breathable and provide good airflow to the skin. Disposable diapers with absorbent cores and a moisture-wicking top layer can help keep your baby's skin dry. If you prefer cloth diapers, ensure they are properly washed and dried to minimize the risk of irritation.

6. Give diaper-free time: Providing your baby with some diaper-free time each day allows their skin to breathe and reduces moisture buildup. Lay a towel or waterproof mat on the floor and let your baby explore and play without a diaper for a short period.

7. Avoid tight diapers or clothing: Diapers or clothing that are too tight can create friction and increase the chances of diaper rash. Ensure the diaper fits snugly but not too tightly, and dress your baby in loose-fitting, breathable clothing.

8. Be cautious with new foods: Introducing new foods to your baby's diet can sometimes result in changes to their bowel movements, which may increase the risk of diaper rash. Monitor their diet and make note of any potential triggers. If you suspect a particular food is causing diaper rash, consult your pediatrician.

9. Be mindful of wipes and detergents: Some babies may have sensitivities or allergies to certain wipes or laundry detergents. If you notice your baby's skin reacting to a specific brand of wipes or detergent, consider switching to a hypoallergenic or fragrance-free alternative.

By following these preventive measures and monitoring your baby's skin regularly, you can significantly reduce the likelihood of diaper rash and help keep your little one comfortable.

BATHING YOUR NEWBORN

Bathing your baby can be a wonderful bonding experience while also keeping them clean and comfortable. Here's a step-by-step guide to help you navigate bathing your newborn:

1. Gather the necessary supplies: Before starting the bath, make sure you have everything you need within reach. This includes a mild baby soap, a soft washcloth or sponge, a towel, clean diapers, clean clothes, a clean diaper, and any other bathing accessories you prefer to use.

2. Choose the right time: Pick a time when you and your baby are both calm and relaxed. Many parents find it helpful to bathe their baby in the morning or early evening when they are alert but not overly tired.

3. Prepare the bath area: It's essential to ensure the bath area is safe and comfortable. If you're using a baby bathtub, place it on a stable surface like a bathroom counter or on the floor. If you're using a regular bathtub, use a non-slip mat to prevent accidents. Fill the tub with a few inches of warm water (around 2-3 inches) to a comfortable

temperature of about 100°F (37°C). Test the water with your elbow or a bath thermometer to ensure it's not too hot or too cold.

4. Undress your baby: Gently undress your baby, removing all their clothing, but leave the diaper on until the end of the bath to prevent accidents. Keep them wrapped in a towel or blanket to keep them warm.

5. Support your baby: With one hand, support your baby's head and neck while using your other hand to hold and guide them into the water. Slowly and carefully lower your baby into the tub, using your arm to support their body in a semi-reclining position.

6. Wash your baby: Wet the washcloth or sponge with warm water and use it to gently clean your baby's body. Start with their face, wiping gently from the forehead down to the chin. Use a little bit of mild baby soap on the cloth to wash their body, starting from the neck and moving down to their chest, arms, belly, legs, and feet. Be sure to clean the diaper area thoroughly.

7. Rinse your baby: Use a cup or your hand to pour warm water gently over your baby's body to rinse off the soap. Take care not to get water in their eyes or ears. Make sure all the soap is rinsed off to avoid any skin irritation.

8. Dry and dress your baby: Lift your baby out of the tub, using a towel to support their head and body. Pat them dry gently, paying attention

to all the skin folds, such as under the neck, in the armpits, and around the diaper area. Once they are dry, apply any necessary creams or lotions recommended by your pediatrician. Then, dress your baby in clean clothes and a fresh diaper.

9. Post-bath care: After bathing, take a few moments to cuddle and bond with your baby. It's also an ideal time to trim their nails if needed and clean their ears using a soft cloth or cotton ball (never insert anything into the ear canal).

Bathing a baby requires extra attention to ensure their safety. Here are some important safety tips to keep in mind while bathing your little one:

1. Never leave your baby unattended: Babies can drown in just a few inches of water, so it's crucial to never leave them alone in the bathtub, even for a moment. If you need to step away, wrap your baby in a towel and take them with you.

2. Maintain a firm grip: Always keep a secure hold on your baby while bathing them. Use one hand to support their head and neck and the other hand to support their body. Babies can be slippery when wet, so maintaining a firm grip is essential.

3. Check the water temperature: Before placing your baby in the water, test the temperature with your elbow or a bath thermometer. The water should be comfortably warm, around

100°F (37°C). It's better to err on the side of slightly cooler water to avoid scalding your baby's delicate skin.

4. Use non-slip mats: Place a non-slip mat or adhesive strips on the bottom of the bathtub to provide stability and prevent slipping. This is especially important if you're using a regular bathtub instead of a baby bathtub.

5. Avoid overfilling the tub: Fill the bathtub with just a few inches of water, enough to cover your baby's body. Too much water can increase the risk of your baby accidentally submerging their face or slipping under the water.

6. Be cautious with bath seats or rings: While some parents use bath seats or rings to help support their baby during bathing, they are not a substitute for close supervision. Always keep your hands on your baby and never rely solely on these devices to prevent accidents.

7. Be mindful of water temperature changes: Babies can be sensitive to sudden changes in water temperature. Avoid exposing them to cold drafts or adding hot water while they are in the tub. If you need to adjust the temperature, do so gradually.

8. Secure toiletries and accessories: Keep all toiletries, such as baby shampoo, soap, and lotions, within arm's reach but out of your

baby's reach. This prevents the risk of your baby accidentally grabbing or ingesting these products.

9. Trim your baby's nails: Babies' nails can be sharp, and they may accidentally scratch themselves while bathing. Regularly trim their nails to prevent any injuries.

10.   Learn infant CPR and first aid: It's always a good idea for parents and caregivers to learn infant CPR and basic first aid techniques. Knowing how to respond in case of an emergency can provide you with the necessary skills and confidence to handle unexpected situations.

By following these safety tips, you can create a secure and enjoyable bathing experience for your baby while minimizing the risk of accidents or injuries.

THE UMBILICAL CORD

The umbilical cord is a vital structure that connects a developing baby to the placenta in the mother's womb. Here's some information to help you understand the umbilical cord:

1. Structure: The umbilical cord is a flexible, rope-like structure that typically measures around 20 inches (50 centimeters) in length

and about half an inch (1-2 centimeters) in diameter. It contains three main components:

a. One vein: The umbilical vein carries oxygenated and nutrient-rich blood from the placenta to the baby, providing essential nourishment for growth and development.

b. Two arteries: The umbilical arteries carry deoxygenated blood and waste products from the baby back to the placenta, where they are eliminated.

2. Development and function: The umbilical cord forms during early pregnancy, around the fifth week of gestation. It acts as a lifeline between the baby and the placenta, serving as a conduit for the exchange of oxygen, nutrients, and waste products. The placenta provides oxygen and nutrients to the baby, while the baby's waste products, such as carbon dioxide, are carried away through the umbilical cord.

3. Protection and insulation: The umbilical cord is surrounded by a jelly-like substance called Wharton's jelly, which provides protection and insulation for the blood vessels within. This jelly-like substance helps prevent compression or damage to the blood vessels, ensuring the uninterrupted flow of blood between the baby and the placenta.

4. Cord clamping and cutting: After the baby is born, healthcare providers typically clamp and cut the umbilical cord. The timing of cord clamping can vary, and there are different approaches, such as delayed cord clamping, where the cord is not clamped immediately after birth but left intact for a short period. Delayed cord clamping has been associated with potential benefits, including increased blood volume and iron stores for the baby.

5. Umbilical cord care after birth: After the umbilical cord is cut, a small stump remains attached to the baby's belly button (navel). Proper care of the umbilical cord stump involves keeping it clean, dry, and exposed to air. It gradually dries out and falls off within one to three weeks, leaving behind a healed belly button.

6. Cord blood banking: The blood within the umbilical cord and placenta contains valuable stem cells that can be collected and stored for potential future use. Cord blood banking is the process of collecting and preserving this blood for possible medical treatments. It is a personal choice and can be discussed with healthcare providers or cord blood banking facilities.

7. Variations and abnormalities: In some cases, the umbilical cord may have variations or abnormalities, such as knots, loops, or additional blood vessels. Most of these variations are harmless and don't cause any complications. However, in rare instances, certain cord abnormalities may lead to complications during

pregnancy or delivery. Healthcare providers closely monitor these situations to ensure the well-being of both the mother and the baby.

It's important to discuss any specific questions or concerns about the umbilical cord with your healthcare provider, as they can provide personalized information and guidance based on your individual circumstances.

Taking care of your baby's umbilical cord stump is an essential part of newborn care. Here are some guidelines to help you with umbilical cord care:

1. Keep the area clean and dry: Keep the umbilical cord stump clean and dry to promote healing and prevent infection. During diaper changes, gently clean around the base of the cord stump with a clean, damp cloth or cotton ball. Pat the area dry with a clean cloth or allow it to air dry.

2. Keep the stump exposed to air: Exposing the umbilical cord stump to air helps it dry out and fall off more quickly. To facilitate this, fold down the top edge of your baby's diaper to keep the stump exposed. Additionally, dress your baby in loose-fitting clothing that doesn't rub against the stump.

3. Avoid covering the stump: It's important not to cover the umbilical cord stump with tight clothing, diapers, or plastic wraps. Allowing air to circulate around the stump helps prevent moisture buildup and speeds up the healing process.

4. Use only water: In most cases, using plain water is sufficient for cleaning the umbilical cord stump. Avoid using soap, alcohol, or any other cleansers unless specifically recommended by your healthcare provider. These products can be harsh and may irritate the sensitive area.

5. Watch for signs of infection: While the umbilical cord stump is healing, it's essential to monitor it for any signs of infection. Contact your healthcare provider if you notice redness, swelling, foul odor, pus, or excessive bleeding around the stump. These may indicate an infection that requires medical attention.

6. Handle with care: When cleaning the umbilical cord stump, be gentle to avoid causing any discomfort or harm to your baby. Use a soft touch and be careful not to pull or tug on the stump.

7. Wait for the stump to fall off naturally: The umbilical cord stump will usually dry up and fall off on its own within one to three weeks after birth. It's important not to try to remove the stump

prematurely, even if it looks like it's ready to come off. Let it detach naturally to minimize the risk of infection.

8. Follow your healthcare provider's advice: Your healthcare provider may have specific instructions or recommendations for umbilical cord care based on your baby's individual circumstances. Always follow their guidance and reach out to them if you have any questions or concerns.

Remember, proper care of the umbilical cord stump helps prevent infection and promotes healing. By keeping the area clean, dry, and exposed to air, you can ensure a healthy transition as your baby's umbilical cord stump naturally falls off.

CHAPTER 6

BABY'S HEALTH AND WELLNESS

Newborn screening is an important part of your baby's healthcare, so it's great that you're seeking information about it. Newborn screening is a set of tests conducted shortly after your baby is born to detect certain genetic, metabolic, and hormonal disorders that may not be apparent at birth but can be treated if identified early. Here's what you need to know:

Purpose: Newborn screening aims to identify conditions that, if left untreated, could cause serious health problems or developmental delays. Early detection and treatment can significantly improve the outcome for affected babies.

Timing: Newborn screening is usually performed within the first 24 to 48 hours after birth. In some cases, additional tests may be conducted at a later stage.

Procedure: A small amount of blood is collected from your baby's heel using a lancet. The blood sample is then sent to a laboratory for analysis. The process is generally quick and simple, and it's done while you're still at the hospital.

Tests: The specific tests included in newborn screening vary from country to country or even between states. However, there are a few common conditions that are screened for worldwide. These typically include:

a. Phenylketonuria (PKU): PKU is an inherited disorder that affects the ability to break down an amino acid called phenylalanine. If left untreated, it can lead to intellectual disability.

b. Hypothyroidism: This condition occurs when the thyroid gland doesn't produce enough thyroid hormones, which are crucial for brain development. Early detection and treatment can prevent complications.

c. Galactosemia: Galactosemia is a disorder that affects the body's ability to process galactose, a sugar found in milk. If untreated, it can lead to serious complications.

d. Sickle cell disease: This is an inherited blood disorder that affects the production of hemoglobin, leading to red blood cell deformities and various health problems.

e. Cystic fibrosis: A genetic disorder that affects the lungs, digestive system, and other organs. Early detection allows for better management and treatment.

Additional conditions: Depending on your location, newborn screening may also include tests for other conditions such as congenital adrenal hyperplasia, hearing loss, or certain metabolic disorders.

Follow-up: If the screening tests indicate a potential issue, further diagnostic testing will be necessary to confirm the diagnosis. In such cases, your healthcare provider will guide you through the next steps, including additional testing, consultation with specialists, and treatment options.

VACCINATION

As a new mum, it's wonderful that you're seeking information about vaccination for your baby. Vaccination is an essential aspect of your child's healthcare and plays a crucial role in protecting them from various infectious diseases. Here's some important information to help educate you about vaccinations for your baby:

1. What are vaccines?

Vaccines are biological substances that stimulate the immune system to recognize and fight against specific diseases. They contain weakened or killed pathogens or pieces of pathogens, such as bacteria or viruses, which help the body develop immunity without causing the actual disease.

2. Why are vaccines important?

Vaccines are vital for protecting your baby from serious and potentially life-threatening diseases. They work by preparing your child's immune system to recognize and fight off specific pathogens. Vaccines have been instrumental in reducing the prevalence of many infectious diseases worldwide and have saved countless lives.

3. Are vaccines safe?

Vaccines undergo rigorous testing and monitoring to ensure their safety and effectiveness. Common side effects are typically mild, such as redness or soreness at the injection site or a low-grade fever. Serious side effects are rare but can occur. However, the risks associated with vaccines are much lower than the risks of developing the diseases they protect against.

4. How does the vaccination schedule work?

Vaccinations are administered in a specific schedule to ensure optimal protection for your baby. The schedule is designed to provide immunity at the earliest possible age while considering the vulnerability of infants to specific diseases. It's crucial to follow the recommended immunization schedule provided by your healthcare provider to ensure your baby receives vaccines at the appropriate times.

5. Herd immunity and its significance:

Vaccination not only protects your baby but also contributes to the concept of herd immunity. When a significant portion of the population is immunized against a disease, it becomes harder for the disease to spread, protecting those who are unable to receive vaccines (e.g., infants too young to be vaccinated or individuals with certain medical conditions). By vaccinating your child, you're also helping protect vulnerable members of your community.

Vaccination schedule

The universal vaccination schedule may vary slightly depending on the country and region. However, this is a general outline of the recommended vaccines and their corresponding ages for infants and children. It's important to consult with your healthcare provider to get the specific schedule applicable to your location. Here is a commonly followed universal vaccination schedule:

Vaccine	Age
BCG	At birth
HEPATITIS B- Birth dose	At birth
OPV-0	At birth
OPV- 1,2&3	At 6 weeks, 10 weeks and 14 weeks
ROTAVIRUS	At 6 weeks, 10 weeks and 14 weeks
IPV	At 6 weeks and 14 weeks
PENTAVALENT 1,2&3	At 6 weeks, 10 weeks and 14 weeks
PCV	At 6 weeks and 14 weeks
MMR- 1st dose	9-12 Months
VITAMIN A- 1st dose	At 9 months

KEYWORDS

OPV- Oral polio vaccine

IPV- inactivated polio vaccine

PCV- pneumococcal conjugate vaccine

PENTAVALENT- Combination of: diphtheria, pertussis, tetanus, hepatitis B

MMR- Measles, mumps, rubella

Please note that this is a general guideline, and the specific schedule may vary depending on your country's recommendations and any additional vaccines that might be recommended for certain high-risk groups. Always consult with your healthcare provider to ensure you have the most accurate and up-to-date information for your baby's vaccination schedule.

It's equally essential to understand the life-threatening diseases that vaccinations can help prevent in your baby. Vaccinations are designed to protect against various infectious diseases, some of which can have severe consequences. Here are a few examples of life-threatening diseases that can be prevented through vaccination:

1. Measles: Measles is a highly contagious viral illness that can lead to serious complications, including pneumonia, encephalitis (inflammation of the brain), and even death, particularly in young children.

2. Polio: Polio is a viral disease that can cause paralysis, leading to permanent disability or even death. Although polio has been largely eliminated in many parts of the world, vaccination is still crucial to ensure complete eradication.

3. Pertussis (Whooping Cough): Pertussis is a bacterial infection that causes severe coughing fits, making it difficult to breathe. It can be life-threatening, especially for infants who are at a higher risk of complications, including pneumonia, seizures, brain damage, and death.

4. Meningococcal Disease: Meningococcal disease is caused by a bacterium and can manifest as meningitis (inflammation of the protective membranes around the brain and spinal cord) or bloodstream infections. It can lead to rapid deterioration, sepsis, organ failure, and death.

5. Pneumococcal Disease: Pneumococcal disease is caused by the bacterium Streptococcus pneumoniae and can lead to severe infections such as pneumonia, meningitis, and bloodstream infections. It poses a significant risk to young children, and vaccination helps protect against these potentially life-threatening conditions.

6. Hepatitis B: Hepatitis B is a viral infection that primarily affects the liver. It can cause chronic liver disease, liver cancer, and even liver

failure. Vaccination against hepatitis B is typically administered shortly after birth to provide early protection.

These are just a few examples, and vaccines also protect against diseases such as diphtheria, tetanus, rotavirus, Haemophilus influenzae type b (Hib), chickenpox (varicella), and others that can cause severe illness or complications in babies and children.

By ensuring your baby receives the recommended vaccinations, you can significantly reduce the risk of these life-threatening diseases. It's important to follow the vaccination schedule recommended by your healthcare provider to provide your child with the best possible protection against these preventable illnesses. Remember, vaccines are a safe and effective way to safeguard your baby's health and well-being.

COMMON ILLNESSES

As a new mum, it's important to familiarize yourself with common illnesses that can affect babies. While it's natural for babies to have occasional health issues, understanding these common illnesses can help you recognize the symptoms, seek appropriate care, and provide comfort to your little one. Here are some of the common illnesses that babies may experience:

1. Common Cold: Babies are susceptible to the common cold, which is caused by different viruses. Symptoms may include a runny or stuffy nose, sneezing, coughing, mild fever, and fussiness. Ensure

your baby stays hydrated, use saline drops to clear nasal congestion, and provide comfort measures such as gentle suctioning and elevating the head.

2. Gastroenteritis (Stomach Bug): Gastroenteritis refers to inflammation of the stomach and intestines, often caused by a viral or bacterial infection. Symptoms include vomiting, diarrhea, stomach cramps, and sometimes a low-grade fever. Keep your baby hydrated with fluids, offer small and frequent feedings, and consult a healthcare provider if symptoms worsen or persist.

3. Diaper Rash: Diaper rash is a common condition characterized by redness, irritation, and soreness in the diaper area. It is often caused by prolonged exposure to moisture, friction, or irritation from urine and feces. Change diapers frequently, keep the area clean and dry, and apply a barrier cream to protect the skin.

4. Thrush: Thrush is a fungal infection caused by the Candida fungus. It commonly affects the mouth and appears as white patches on the tongue, gums, or inner cheeks. It may cause discomfort during feeding. Consult a healthcare provider for appropriate antifungal treatment.

5. Ear Infections: Ear infections are common in babies and are usually caused by bacterial or viral infections. Symptoms may include ear pain, tugging at the ears, irritability, fever, and

difficulty sleeping. Consult a healthcare provider for diagnosis and appropriate treatment.

6. Rashes: Babies may develop various types of rashes, such as diaper rash, heat rash, eczema, or allergic reactions. The appearance and cause of the rash can vary. Consult a healthcare provider for an accurate diagnosis and guidance on treatment and management.

If your baby shows severe symptoms, has a high fever, difficulty breathing, or if you're concerned about their health, always seek medical attention promptly. Your healthcare provider will be able to provide a proper diagnosis and recommend the appropriate treatment for your baby's specific condition.

SAFETY MEASURES

Ensuring a safe environment is crucial for your baby's well-being. As a mum, it's important to take proactive measures to create a safe and child-friendly home. Here are some key safety measures to consider:

1. Babyproofing: Babyproofing involves making your home safe by identifying potential hazards and taking steps to minimize them. Install safety gates at the top and bottom of stairs, use safety latches on cabinets and drawers, secure heavy furniture and electronics to prevent tipping, and cover electrical outlets with

outlet covers. Also, keep small objects, choking hazards, and toxic substances out of reach.

2. Crib Safety: Follow safe sleep practices for your baby. Use a crib that meets safety standards, with a firm mattress and fitted sheet. Remove pillows, blankets, stuffed animals, and other soft objects from the crib to reduce the risk of suffocation. Position your baby on their back to sleep.

3. Kitchen Safety: Keep hazardous items, such as cleaning supplies and sharp objects, locked away or out of reach in locked cabinets. Use stove knob covers to prevent accidental burns or injuries. Never leave your baby unattended in the kitchen, especially when cooking.

4. Bathroom Safety: Keep the bathroom door closed and consider installing a toilet lock to prevent drowning hazards. Store medications, toiletries, and cleaning products in locked cabinets. Set the water heater temperature below 120°F (49°C) to avoid scalding.

5. Window Safety: Install window guards or window stops to prevent falls. Ensure windows cannot be opened more than a few inches to prevent your baby from crawling or falling through.

6. Cord Safety: Keep cords from blinds, curtains, and electronics out of your baby's reach. Use cord winders or cord shorteners to prevent strangulation hazards.

7. Smoke and Carbon Monoxide Detectors: Install smoke detectors on each level of your home and near sleeping areas. Test them regularly and change batteries as needed. Consider installing carbon monoxide detectors, especially near sleeping areas and fuel-burning appliances.

8. Secure Rugs and Flooring: Use non-slip pads or rugs with non-slip backing to prevent slips and falls. Secure loose cords or wires along the walls or use cord covers.

9. Supervision and Awareness: Always supervise your baby and be aware of their surroundings. Be cautious of open windows, hot beverages, sharp objects, and potential hazards both inside and outside the home.

10. Emergency Preparedness: Keep emergency numbers readily available. Learn infant and child CPR and basic first aid techniques. First aid techniques will be discussed below.

Stay vigilant and adapt your safety measures as your baby grows and becomes more mobile. Regularly reassess your home for potential risks and make necessary adjustments to maintain a safe environment for your little one.

FIRST AID BASICS

As a new mum, having a basic understanding of first aid can be invaluable in managing common injuries or emergencies that may occur with your baby. While it's important to seek professional medical help for serious or life-threatening situations, knowing some first aid basics can help you provide immediate care. Here are a few key first aid principles and skills to consider:

1. CPR (Cardiopulmonary Resuscitation): CPR is a lifesaving technique used to revive someone who is not breathing or whose heart has stopped. Learning infant CPR is highly recommended. Consider taking a certified CPR course that includes infant CPR to gain hands-on training and confidence in performing this procedure correctly.

2. Choking: Babies have a tendency to put objects in their mouths, making them prone to choking. If your baby is conscious and choking, perform infant choking first aid by delivering back blows and chest thrusts. If the baby becomes unconscious, start CPR immediately.

3. Burns: Immediately cool a burn with cool (not cold) running water for at least 10 minutes to reduce the temperature and severity of the burn. Remove any clothing or jewelry near the burn area, but do not peel away any stuck fabric. For severe burns, seek medical attention.

4. Cuts and Scrapes: Clean minor cuts and scrapes with mild soap and water. Apply gentle pressure with a clean cloth or sterile gauze to stop any bleeding. Apply an antiseptic ointment and cover with a sterile adhesive bandage or dressing.

5. Falls: If your baby falls, observe them closely for signs of injury or unusual behavior. Apply a cold compress or ice pack wrapped in a cloth to any areas that are swollen or bruised. If you suspect a serious head or neck injury, do not move your baby and seek immediate medical attention.

6. Allergic Reactions: If your baby displays signs of an allergic reaction, such as difficulty breathing, swelling of the face or lips, or a rash, seek medical help immediately. If your baby has been prescribed an epinephrine auto-injector (e.g., EpiPen), be familiar with how to use it as directed by your healthcare provider.

7. Fever: If your baby has a fever, follow the guidelines provided by your healthcare provider. Acetaminophen or ibuprofen may be recommended in appropriate doses for babies over a certain age, but always consult with your healthcare provider before giving any medication.

Having basic first aid knowledge and being prepared can help you respond calmly and effectively in emergencies while waiting for professional medical assistance to arrive.

DEALING WITH A FUSSY BABY

Handling a fussy baby can be challenging, but with patience and understanding, you can help soothe and calm your little one. Here are some tips to help you navigate those fussy moments:

1. Check Basic Needs: Assess if your baby is hungry, needs a diaper change, or is tired. Addressing these basic needs can often help alleviate fussiness.

2. Comfort and Cuddle: Hold your baby close and provide gentle rocking or swaying motions. The feeling of security and warmth can help soothe them. You can also try babywearing using a carrier or sling.

3. Create a Calming Environment: Dim the lights, reduce noise levels, and create a calm and peaceful atmosphere. Some babies find white noise or gentle music soothing. Experiment with different sounds or use a shushing sound to mimic the womb environment.

4. Use Swaddling: Swaddling can help provide a sense of security and limit their startle reflex. Wrap your baby firmly in a

lightweight blanket, ensure their hips and legs have room to move.

5. Offer a Pacifier: Pacifiers can help satisfy your baby's need to suck and provide comfort. If you are breastfeeding your baby, wait until breastfeeding is well-established before introducing a pacifier.

6. Try Gentle Massage: Use gentle strokes and soft pressure to massage your baby's back, tummy, or limbs. This will aid the relaxation of their muscles and promote a sense of calm.

7. Experiment with Different Positions: Hold your baby in different positions, such as upright against your shoulder or cradled in your arms. Some babies may find certain positions more soothing than others.

8. Engage in Gentle Movement: Sometimes, rhythmic movements can help calm a fussy baby. You can try walking around the room, taking a car ride, or using a baby swing or bouncer.

9. Offer Distractions: Use age-appropriate toys or objects with different textures, colors, or sounds to distract and engage your baby's attention. This can help redirect their focus and provide some relief.

10.   Stay Calm and Patient: Babies can pick up on your energy, so try to remain calm and patient. Take deep breaths, speak softly, and provide a reassuring presence. Remember that fussiness is normal and temporary.

11.   Take Breaks: If you're feeling overwhelmed or frustrated, it's okay to take short breaks. Place your baby in a safe space, such as a crib or bassinet, and give yourself a few minutes to collect yourself before returning to soothe them.

It's important to note that each baby is unique, and what works for one may not work for another. Be open to trying different techniques and strategies until you find what helps soothe your baby. Trust your instincts and seek support from your healthcare provider, a lactation consultant, or experienced parents if you need additional guidance or reassurance.

CHAPTER 7

SELF CARE FOR THE NEW MOTHER

As a new mum, it's natural to prioritize your baby's needs, but it's equally important to prioritize your own well-being. Taking care of yourself physically, mentally, and emotionally is essential for your overall health and ability to care for your baby. Here are some key considerations for prioritizing your well-being:

1. Self-Care: Make time for self-care activities that you enjoy and find rejuvenating. It can be as simple as taking a relaxing bath, reading a book, going for a walk, practicing mindfulness or meditation, or engaging in hobbies. Remember, self-care isn't selfish—it's necessary for your well-being.

2. Rest and Sleep: Adequate rest and sleep are crucial for your physical and mental health. Try to prioritize sleep by taking naps when your baby sleeps and asking for support from your partner, family, or friends to allow for uninterrupted sleep.

3. Nutrition and Hydration: Maintain a balanced and nutritious diet to fuel your body and support your energy levels. Stay hydrated

by drinking plenty of water throughout the day. Remember to prioritize regular meals and healthy snacks, even when you're busy caring for your baby.

4. Exercise: Engage in regular physical activity that suits your postpartum condition and is approved by your healthcare provider. Exercise can boost your energy levels, reduce stress, and improve your overall well-being. Consider activities such as walking, postnatal yoga, or pelvic floor exercises.

5. Social Support: Connect with other new moms or join support groups to share experiences, seek advice, and find emotional support. Building a network of supportive individuals can provide a sense of community and help reduce feelings of isolation.

6. Seek Help: Don't hesitate to ask for help when you need it. Reach out to your partner, family members, or friends to assist with baby care or household tasks. Delegate responsibilities to create time for self-care or to seek professional help if needed.

7. Emotional Well-being: Pay attention to your emotional health and seek help if you experience symptoms of postpartum depression or anxiety. Reach out to your healthcare provider or a mental health professional for guidance and support.

8. Time Management: Prioritize and manage your time effectively. Create a schedule that balances your baby's needs with your own

activities and responsibilities. It's important to find a routine that works for you and allows for time dedicated to self-care.

Taking care of yourself doesn't mean neglecting your baby—it means ensuring that you are in the best possible physical and mental state to provide the care and support your baby needs. By prioritizing your well-being, you can better navigate the joys and challenges of motherhood and foster a positive and healthy environment for both you and your baby.

COMMON POSTPARTUM CHALLENGES

After giving birth, many mothers experience various postpartum challenges as their bodies recover and adjust to the demands of motherhood. It's important to be aware of these common challenges and know that you're not alone. Here are some postpartum challenges that mothers often face:

1. Physical Recovery: Your body needs time to heal after childbirth. You may experience discomfort, pain, or soreness in the perineal area (if you had a vaginal delivery) or from a cesarean section incision. You might also have breast engorgement, sore nipples, or changes in urination and bowel movements. Give yourself time to rest, follow your healthcare provider's recommendations for pain management, and reach out for support if needed.

2. Hormonal Changes: Hormonal shifts after childbirth can lead to mood swings, irritability, weepiness, or the "baby blues." These feelings are normal and typically resolve within a few weeks. However, if you are having constant feelings of sadness, agitation or depression, it could be a sign of postpartum depression, and it's important to seek professional help.

3. Sleep Deprivation: Adjusting to your baby's sleep patterns can be challenging, leading to sleep deprivation. Insomnia (lack of sleep or insufficient sleep) due to child care can affect your mood, energy levels, and your general well-being. Try to rest when your baby sleeps, accept help from others, and establish a sleep routine that works for you and your baby.

4. Breastfeeding Challenges: Breastfeeding can be both rewarding and challenging. Many mothers face issues such as sore nipples, engorgement, low milk supply, or difficulties with latching. Seek support from a lactation consultant, attend breastfeeding support groups, or consult your healthcare provider for guidance and assistance.

5. Body Image and Self-Esteem: Adjusting to changes in your body postpartum can be emotionally challenging. It's normal to feel self-conscious or struggle with body image. Give yourself time to adjust and focus on self-care and self-acceptance. Surround

yourself with supportive people who understand and value your journey as a mother.

6. Time Management and Prioritization: Balancing the demands of caring for a newborn with other responsibilities can be overwhelming. It's important to manage your time effectively and prioritize tasks. Don't hesitate to ask for help from your partner, family, or friends, and be kind to yourself if you can't get everything done.

7. Relationship Changes: The arrival of a baby can bring significant changes to your relationship dynamics. Communication, patience, and understanding are key. Make time for regular communication with your partner, and seek support from each other during this transition period.

8. Feeling Overwhelmed: Motherhood can be overwhelming, and it's common to feel a range of emotions, including anxiety and stress. Reach out to your support system, join motherhood support groups, or consider talking to a therapist who specializes in postpartum issues.

Remember, every mother's experience is unique. If you're facing challenges that significantly impact your well-being or ability to care for yourself and your baby, don't hesitate to seek professional help. Your healthcare provider can provide guidance, support, and appropriate resources to address your specific needs.

ADJUSTING TO YOUR SOCIAL LIFE AFTER CHILDBIRTH

Adjusting to your social life after childbirth can be a significant transition. As a new mum, it's normal to experience changes in your social interactions and routines. Here are some tips to help you navigate this adjustment:

1. Set Realistic Expectations: Recognize that your social life may change for a while as you focus on caring for your baby. Understand that it's okay to prioritize your baby's needs and take time for yourself during this period.

2. Communicate with Loved Ones: Talk openly with your partner, family, and friends about your needs and limitations. Let them know that your availability may be different now, but you still value their support and connection. Establish clear boundaries and communicate your preferences regarding visitors and social activities.

3. Start Small: Begin by gradually reintroducing social activities into your routine. Start with short outings or visits with close friends or family members. This can help you regain confidence and slowly adjust to being out and about with your baby.

4. Join Parenting Groups or Classes: Consider joining local parenting groups, support groups, or classes tailored to new parents. Connecting with other parents who are going through similar experiences can provide a sense of community and understanding. You can share advice, concerns, and joys while building new friendships.

5. Utilize Online Communities: Take advantage of online platforms and forums for connecting with other parents. Virtual communities provide an opportunity to engage with a wide range of parents, exchange experiences, and seek advice without leaving the comfort of your home.

6. Plan Social Outings: Organize outings or meetups with friends who understand and accommodate the needs of your baby. This could involve meeting at baby-friendly locations or planning activities that allow you to socialize while still attending to your baby's needs.

7. Be Flexible: Understand that plans may need to change due to your baby's schedule or needs. Practice flexibility and adaptability when it comes to social engagements. Consider organizing activities that can be easily adjusted or rescheduled if necessary.

8. Take Care of Yourself: Prioritize self-care, including maintaining your physical and mental well-being. Taking time for yourself and

engaging in activities that recharge you can positively impact your social interactions and overall happiness.

Adjusting to your social life takes time, and it's normal to feel a mix of emotions during this period. Trust yourself and your instincts as you navigate this new phase of life. With patience, open communication, and a supportive network, you can gradually find a balance that works for you and your baby.